THE CHOCOLATE CONTROVERSY

The Bad, the Mediocre and the Awesome

Holly Fourchalk, PhD, DNM®, RHT, HT

CHOICES UNLIMITED
FOR
HEALTH & WELLNESS

Choices Unlimited for Health & Wellness
Dr. Holly Fourchalk, Ph.D., DNM®, RHT, HT
Tel: 604.764.5203
Fax: 604.465.7964
Website: www.choicesunlimited.ca
E-mail: holly@choicesunlimited.ca

Editing, Interior Design and Cover Design: Wendy
Dewar Hughes, Summer Bay Press

ISBN: 978-1-927626-01-6
Digital ISBN: 978-1-927626-02-3

To my Parents

For all their support and encouragement
My Dad for his ever listening ear
My mother for her open mind

THE CHOCOLATE CONTROVERSY

CONTENTS

ONE

Why do we love chocolate?

Chocolate has a long history. Historically, chocolate was considered a food from the gods. It was used in rituals, for royalty, to protect warriors going into battle, and of course, as an aphrodisiac. The chocolate of the 1900's became an entirely different "food" than chocolate of the ages.

Why has it been used so extensively, and why do we like it so much? Well, that probably has to do, in part, with how nutritious it is for the body.

Perhaps it truly is a food from the gods as it has a significant impact on everything in the body, including:

- Autoimmune Disease
- Bone Density
- Brain function and both emotional and

cognitive challenges
- Diabetes
- Gut and food absorption
- Heart and cardiovascular disease
- Inflammatory disease
- Liver and detox
- Skin and healthy hair and nails
- Weight management

Throughout history, people have enjoyed fruit. Fruits are full of wonderful substances like polyphenols, anti-oxidants, vitamins, minerals, soluble and non-soluble fibers, and more. Chocolate, though not technically a fruit, is no exception.

But somehow chocolate is different. Why? It is a food that:

- tastes great
- feels great in the mouth
- is an aphrodisiac
- provides natural anti-depressants
- provides endorphins
- provides energy
- is full of nutrients that the body requires.

It has to be different!

This book will explore the history of the chocolate plant; the development of the chocolate food; the detriments of chocolate and most importantly, the benefits of chocolate.

There is a wide distribution of "choc-aholics" around the world with Switzerland in the lead consuming about 19 pounds of chocolate per person per year, according to David Wolfe & Shazzie's Naked Chocolate. Belgians, Dutch, Germans and Austrians fall in behind consuming about 14 pounds of chocolate per year. I have not read anywhere where Canadians and Americans fall on this scale but the Japanese fall way behind with about 3 pounds per person.

Our delight with chocolate has even provided the backdrop for several movies like, Willie Wonka and The Chocolate Factory (1971); Four and a Half Women a.k.a. Chocolate for Breakfast (1998); Chocolat (2000); Charlie & the Chocolate Factory (2005); Chocolate Lessons (2007); In Search of the Heart of Chocolate

(2008); and more movies in languages other than English – yes, we do love our chocolate.

Myths & Misconceptions about Chocolate

Science has conclusively proven the following myths and misconceptions about chocolate are wrong:

1) "Chocolate is addictive." Cacao is not in any way physically addictive.

2) "Chocolate has caffeine." Cacao does not naturally contain any caffeine. It does have a caffeine-like molecule that does stimulate caffeinic receptors but does so differently than caffeine.

3) "I am allergic to chocolate." A true chocolate or cocoa allergy is rare even though many people claim to be allergic to it. A study shows that only one out of every 500 people who thought they were allergic to chocolate actually tested positive.

4) "Chocolate causes acne." Cacao does not promote acne. Most researchers to-day believe acne to be more connected

with lifestyle (stress) and hormones than any food at all. Cacao has been proven to have no effect on acne, positive or negative. Usually when people make this claim they are talking about the sugar in candy, not the cacao, although a link between sugar and acne has also never been proven.

5) "Chocolate makes you fat." Cacao does not promote obesity in any way. (Although the sugar and wax in candy bars does!) Cocoa Butter is an unsaturated fat like olive oil or avocado and has shown no ill health effects whatsoever and, in fact, is very beneficial.

6) "Chocolate rots your teeth." Cacao does not promote tooth decay (although the sugar in candy bars does!) In fact, pure chocolate actually helps prevent tooth decay and some societies have used cocoa butter to coat the teeth in order to protect them.

Myths about chocolate which may have some truth to them:

"Chocolate causes headaches."

Theobromide is a powerful stimulant and it is not uncommon for people to have reactions such as headaches when ingesting a stimulant.

I have been attempting to test it to cure migraines (opposite of a headache), with some possibly promising results.

Cacao has never been proven to be an aphrodisiac, however

1. Theobromide is proven to cause both physical and mental relaxation, a sense of well-being and alertness which could certainly promote sexual interest.

2. Chocolate is a "treat"; something most people enjoy. This feeling has proven aphrodisiac effects.

3. For many centuries, chocolate has been identified with love, and yes, with sex. We can react to social identifications whether there is a basis in science or not.

See: http://www.xocoatl.org/science.htm

The following chapters will explore:

- the history of chocolate
- the actual plant and fruit
- the processing of different chocolates
- why chocolate is bad for you
- why chocolate is good for you

We will also explore the science behind the impact real chocolate has on a variety of diseases, disorders, and dysfunctions in the body.

TWO

History of Chocolate

Chocolate's history is as varied as the nutrients it contains.

The cultivation of chocolate and the use of chocolate both as a food and as a medicine, date back to 2000 B.C. in Honduras. Chocolate is also well known throughout many different cultures.

Where the chocolate fascination began is very controversial. Archaeological sites on the Pacific side of Mexico depict evidence of cocoa beverages that were probably fermented, i.e., an alcoholic beverage.

From the Olmecs to the Mayans; from Africa to Central America – cultures have utilized the cacao fruit in ceremonies, rituals and feasts.

Chocolate has a medicinal history as well. It

has been utilized for:

- Stomach issues
- Intestinal issues
- Infections
- Fever
- Coughs
- General nourishment – both as a drink and a food.

An old list of medicinal uses for chocolate included the following:

Medicinal Uses: (including the Seeds, Fruit, Leaves and Bark)

Actions

- Antiseptic
- Cardiotonic
- Diuretic
- Dentifrice
- Emmenagogue
- Parasiticide
- Vasodilator
- Vulnerary
  Can be used in cases of
- Alopecia

- Burn
- Cough
- Dry-Lip
- Eczema
- Eye Conditions
- Headache
- High Blood Pressure
- Kidney Conditions
- Listlessness
- Parturition
- Pilatory
- Rheumatism
- Sarna
- Snake Bite
- Wounds

NOTE:

This is not intended to suggest that Chocolate has all of these medicinal properties but rather that parts of the Cacao plant (possibly including the seeds) if prepared correctly by an expert will have these properties. There are many excellent ethnobotany resources on the web.

See: http://www.xocoatl.org/science.htm

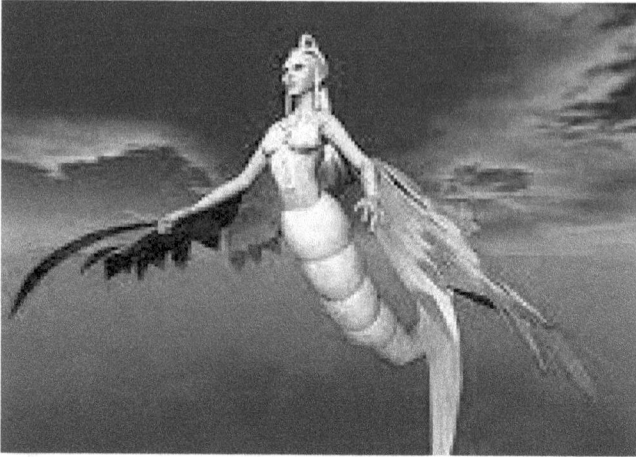

In the last decade, science has really extended this list, as you will see in the following chapters.

The Mayans claim that their God, Heart of Sky, made man from a variety of natural components: water, earth, wood, corn, fruits and cacao. Thus, according to the Maya, we have cacao as part of our natural make-up!

Another historical story from the first century A.D. comes from Central America. The story claims that a revered and respected Mesoamerican deity called Quetzacoatl (Feathered Serpent), not only brought cocoa from the Garden of Life to Earth, but also taught people medicine and how to grow cacao.

Cacao beans became both a valuable commodity and a major form of currency and tribute payment in the Aztec empire (A.D. 1376-1520). A special government official regulated the weights and measures of cacao. He would make sure the price matched the quality of the fruit. Aztec female market vendors prepared the chocolate.

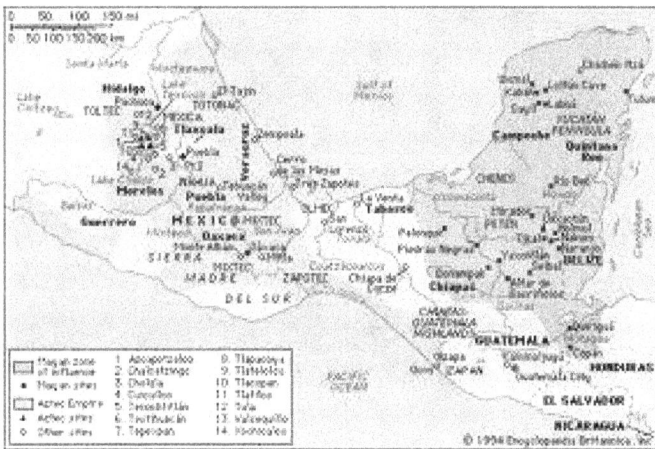

<u>Florentine Codex</u> by Fray Bernardino de Sahagún (1499-1590) is utilized as a main source on Aztec life in the 1500s. The book describes the production of a fine chocolate beverage, "the drink of nobles" infused with chili water, flowers, vanilla, and honey.

The Aztecs knew how to harvest, ferment, roast and grind the cacao seeds. They then mixed the seeds with water, chili peppers, cornmeal and other ingredients. This made a spicy, frothy, chocolate drink. Xocolatl, the term the Aztecs used for chocolate, means "bitter drink".

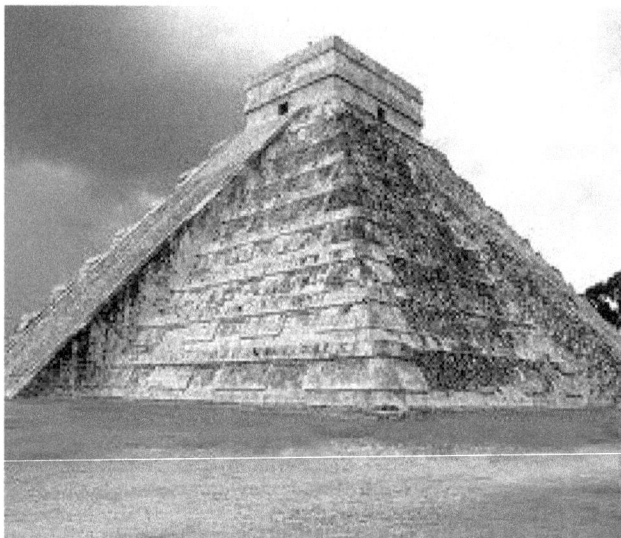

Europeans were introduced to cacao with Christopher Columbus in the early 1500s and again with Cortes when he encountered in the Aztecs. Chocolate as a commodity quickly spread through Europe. The Spanish developed cacao plantations in the Philippines while the French developed plantations in the Caribbean. In 1753 the Swedish scientist, Carl von Linnaeus, named the genus and species. He named the tree Theobroma cacao which translates to "food of the gods".

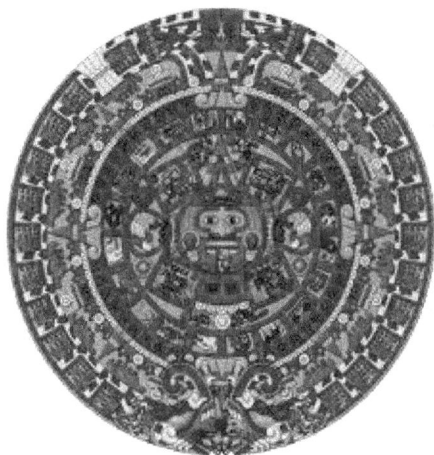

It wasn't long before the Spanish Catholic Church recognized chocolate for both its energy and it's restorative capacity. This effect is somewhat due to theobromine.

Theobromine is a "caffeine-like" molecule that has as impact on the caffeinic receptors in the brain – although it creates a different response than caffeine. Consequently, although this contributes to the energy people get from chocolate, it is very different than the spiking kind of energy that comes from the caffeine in coffee and energy drinks.

The chocolate drink was originally used during periods of fasting. While solids were not allowed in the fast, the nutrient dense drink kept everyone going well.

It is believed that the Spaniards transformed the Aztec term xocolatl – a cold bitter drink with vanilla and spices – into the modern term, chocolate. However, there is still some controversy with that version of history. In due course, the Spaniards enslaved the Mesoamericans to produce cacao and so they could send it back to Spain.

It wasn't just the church and the Spaniards that found chocolate enticing. It didn't take long before the English, Dutch and French began to colonize new areas developing cacao plantations in the cacao-growing lands near the equator.

Britain established plantations in Ceylon (Sri Lanka). Holland established plantations in Venezuela, Java, and Sumatra. France established plantations in the West Indies.

Before long, efforts of these countries resulted in the shipping of cacao to markets back home. Chocolate rapidly became a high demand product.

Sir Hans Sloane (1660 - 1753) was a physician, scientist and the president of the Royal College of Physicians (1727-1741). He had quite the resume (CV). He was appointed Physician Extraordinary to Queen Anne in 1696, George I in 1716 and Physician in Ordinary to George II in 1727. He was also well known for his collections of plants, animals, antiquities and chocolate.

Perhaps his most exciting achievement was coming up with a new recipe for chocolate. When in Jamaica, Sir Sloane was introduced to cocoa as a drink but found it to be nauseating. He took the then expensive and exotic sugar and mixed it with the chocolate creating a sweet drink. Then he went a step further with his recipe and, rather than mixing the sweet chocolate with water, he mixed it with milk. Thus, we have the beginnings of what we now know as milk chocolate!

Initially Sir Sloane's recipe was sold in apothecaries as a medicine. Later, the recipe was sold to the Cadbury brothers in 1897.

The United States, in their rebellion against the British and anything that the British stood for, and after the Boston Tea Party, they took to drinking coffee and chocolate bevereages rather than tea.

Subsequently, wax was introduced into the recipe then high fructose corn syrup, lecithin, vegetable oil, commercial shortening and more.

It was no longer a food of the gods but had become instead, a man-made food. As with any other food, it seems the more man gets involved with processing it, the more harmful it becomes.

THREE

Chocolate – the Plant

The cacao tree belongs to the Theobromoa genus (of which there are approximately 22 species) and belongs to the Sterculiaceae family which includes the African cola nut. It has now been re-classified to the Melvaceae family, i.e., the mallow family that consists of jute, marshmallow, kola nut, baobabs, okra and cotton.

While the most commonly known species of chocolate is the Theobromoa cacao it has apparently been divided into subspecies. The South American species, Theobromoa spaerocarpum, that is a fairly smooth melon like fruit, and the Mesoamerican species, Theobromoa cacao, that is ridged and elongated. Today there are three main varieties: Criollo, Forastero and a combination of the two – Trinitario.

There are different conflicting perspectives on how the cacao tree spread. The oldest theory is that wild cacao was distributed from southeastern Mexico to the Amazon basin. Newer theories claim that cacao originated in the Amazon and was subsequently distributed throughout Central America and Mesoamerica.

See:
(http://www.icco.org/faq/51-cocoa-trees/114-what-is-the-origin-of-the-cocoa-tree.html)

Criollo, the ridged variety, apparently originated in Central America and comes in red, yellow or blue (the blue variety is also referred to as Theobromoa aromica). This species is noted for its rich taste and aroma. It is also more susceptible to disease, ripens late and represents about 5% of the world's chocolate crop.

The Amazonian Theobromoa forastero is a much more durable plant. It has a better capacity to ward off disease, matures quickly, has a high fat content, and provides about 80% of the world's chocolate.

The hybrid Theobromoa trinitario, dates back to the 1800s in Trinidad. It has the more delicate aroma of the Criollo but fosters the more robust nature of the Forastero.

Chocolate – the tree

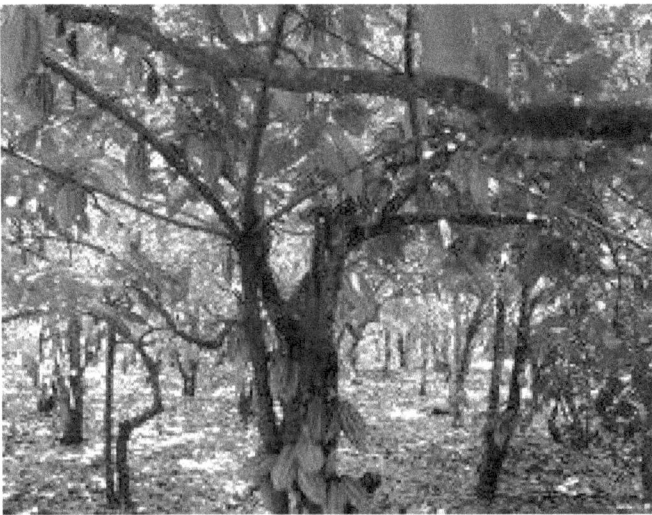

The tree itself grows upwards between 3-10 meters in height, although it begins to branch near the ground. The leaves are somewhat similar to an avocado leaf, growing about 10-25 cm long and 5-8 cm wide. The tree produces flowers and fruit all year long. The flowers have 5 petals and grow straight out of the trunk.

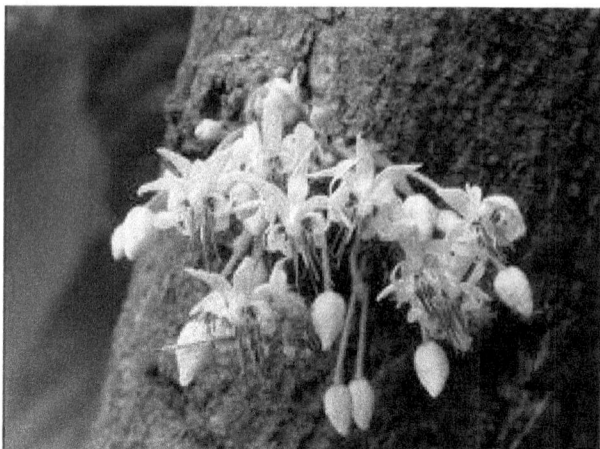

Chocolate – the fruit

The cacao fruit is a pod-like fruit. While it starts off green in color, it evolves into red, orange, yellow, blue or purple colors depending on the variety. The almond shaped fruit grows to about 20 cm in length.

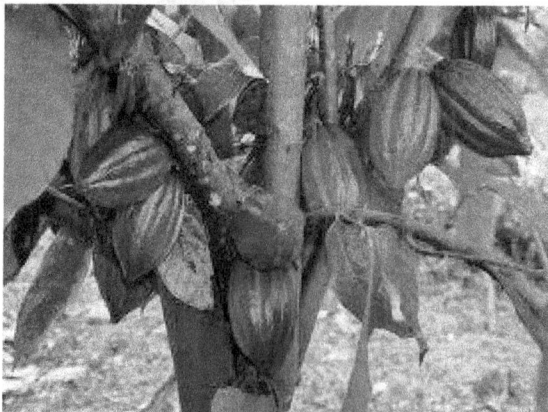

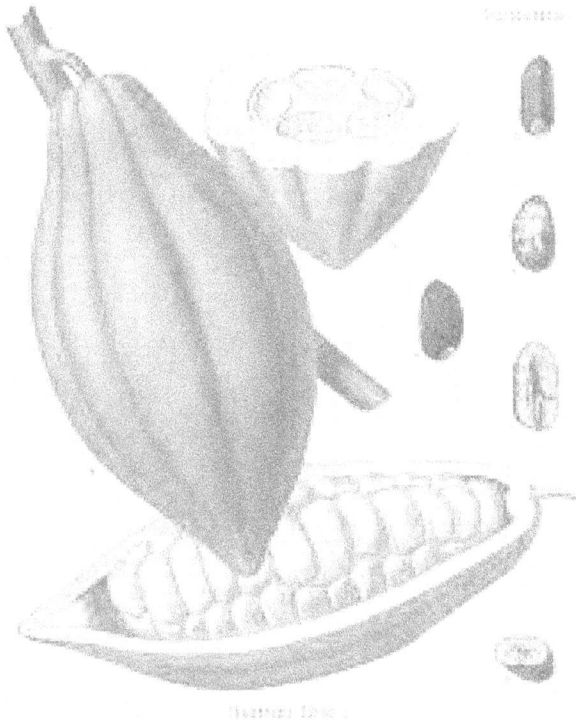

Each particular species has a different number of almond sized seeds within the fruit – some as few as 8-10, others upwards of 60.

These trees are easily adaptable to a wide range of conditions in the tropics. They tend to grow within a mile of the equator and require fairly constant temperatures but they can grow from subtropical dry to very wet tropical zones. They tolerate wind well but thrive with high humidity and regular rainfall conditions.

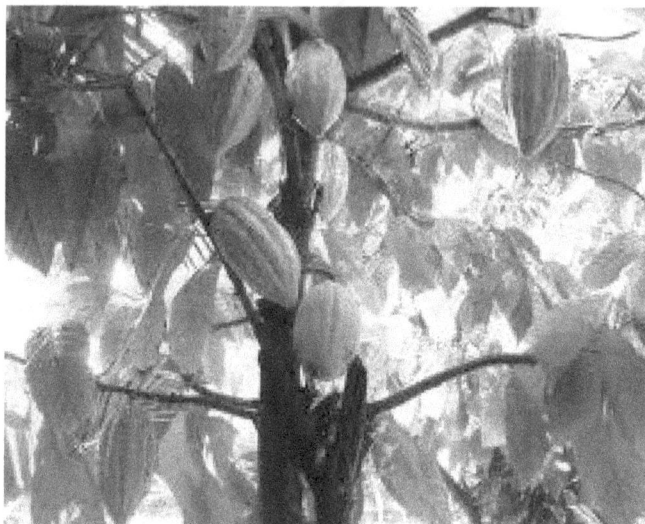

See:
http://www.medicin
ehunter.com/the-
chocolate-tree

The trees tend to prefer shaded areas and are consequent-ly grown with other trees, like rubber, banana, coconut

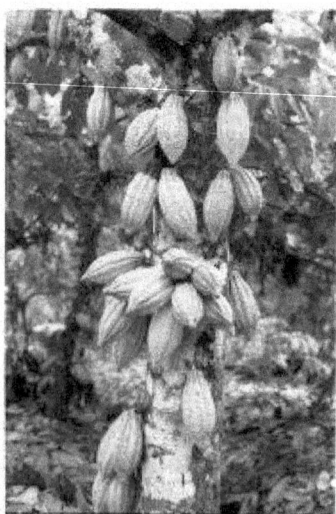

and other palm trees.

Today, cacao is grown in the Ivory Coast, Ghana, Indonesia, Brazil, Cameroon, Caribbean, Malaysia and the Pacific Islands.

FOUR

How Chocolate is Grown and Processed

How chocolate gets from the tree to your mouth and retains its nutritive qualities is hugely important. The manner in which chocolate is cultivated, harvested and processed all play a part in determining whether chocolate has all the nutrients you require.

GENUS

As noted previously, the cocoa plant belongs to the genus Theobroma. Theobroma cacao which is latin for "food of the gods" was recently reclassified under the Malvaceae family, i.e., the mallow family which includes jute, marshmallow, kola nut, okra and cotton.

See:
http://www.kew.org/plants-fungi/Theobroma-cacao.htm

CULTIVATION

There is a vast difference between non-organic, organic and wild crafted plants. When a crop is cultivated, it is planted in rows. It may be planted along with other plants for a given reason, i.e., chocolate is usually planted along with banana trees or palm trees because the chocolate trees need to be in the shade.

We all know that if the cultivated food products are sprayed with pesticides, herbicides, insecticides, etc., the plants absorb these toxic chemicals. These chemicals are then carried to our digestive systems. In addition, the depleted soils used in crop production are frequently enhanced with fertilizers that can also be toxic to us.

Typically, as we become more aware of the affects of toxins in our bodies, we begin to look for organic foods, foods grown without all the added toxic chemicals. These are far better for us. Many farmers are now finding that they have higher yields when they do not use the extra chemicals. This is good news.

However, when plants are cultivated they lose a lot of naturally-occurring nutrients. Just think for a minute of a rich tropical jungle. In the jungle, there is a continual cycling of growth and death. The death and natural composting of all the plants (and animals and microbes) contribute back to the soils making the soils rich with all the nutrients the plant requires. The plant then subsequently gives us the nutrients.

In addition, because the plant in the jungle has to naturally force off all those other microbes they develop strong, healthy immune systems – which they then provide us with.

When chocolate is claimed to be "organic", that's a good thing but if it is "wild crafted" then it is awesome!

HARVESTING

When the fruit is picked, the seeds are removed and dried. Initially, they are covered by a bitter sweet white pulp. When dried and fermented in the sun, the seeds turn a brownish red and these are what are known as the cocoa beans. How long these seeds are dried and the temperatures at which they are dried both have a bearing on the nutrient held in the seed.

See:
http://www.kew.org/plants-fungi/Theobroma-cacao.htm

PROCESSING

The next step in chocolate production is also crucial. Historically, the seeds were ground into a paste. However, in the last century man started pasteurizing foods.

Initially, pasteurization was developed to slow the spoilage of beer, due to microbial growth then the process was applied to dairy (for taxing purposes). Following that, pasteurization was applied to other foods, including chocolate.

As with anything else that is pasteurized, we lose the vast majority of nutrients in the process, i.e., like milk. The reason pasteurized foods have such a long shelf life is that they have no microbes or nutrients to go bad.

Today, sailors will take white bread on their trips – as it will last the longest, i.e., no nutrient to go bad. Likewise, most store-bought chocolate has a long shelf life because there are no nutrients in it.

For now though, let's get back to the cacao seeds. These seeds can be stored for months in cloth sacks before any further processing is done.

The flavor and aroma of chocolate can vary as widely as wines and coffees. A significant part of this variation is determined by the manufacturer. Initially the beans are cleaned through strainers called riddles and then they are roasted. After cooling, they are put into the cracking machines where the bitter outer shells are broken. The inner pieces, called the nibs, are ground into a fine cocoa paste.

The grinding heats up the cocoa butter which may contribute up to 50% of the volume. The cocoa butter is a rich fatty liquid called the chocolate liquor.

This cocoa butter or liquor can be heated and further removed. At this point, various substances are added to the remaining powder, like potassium carbonate which alkalizes the powder and changes how the solid nibs react to liquids such as water or milk. Other components added to the cocoa nibs/solids or butter, may include sugar, lecithin or vanilla.

The chocolate is then both cooled and heated again to stabilize the fat crystals in the chocolate.

See:
http://www.medicinehunter.com/the-chocolate-tree

While this identifies the most common procedures utilized with chocolate, there are a few variations such as dutch pressing or Xocai® processing. Xocai® has a special patent that protects all the anti-oxidants and other nutrients in chocolate. The more heat that is applied, the higher the loss of nutrients, especially with regard to the anti-oxidants which are sensitive to heat.

FIVE

Why is Chocolate Bad for You?

Old Beliefs:

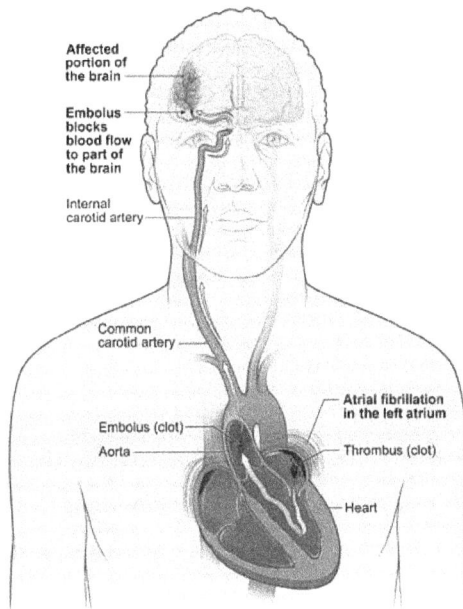

People believe that chocolate is a junk food and therefore it is bad for you. Unfortunately, as we know from chapter one, man did turn this "food of the gods" into a junk food.

When man pasteurizes food (cooked between temperatures of 160-200 degrees Fahrenheit) the microbes are eliminated. In addition, the molecules/nutrients become "denatured". This means that the nutrients are structurally changed.

We have enzymes to break down and metabolize nutrients in their natural form but when the nutrients are "denatured" or structurally changed, we no longer have the required enzymes to metabolize them and they become toxic to the body.

In addition, when we add waxes and high fructose corn syrup:

- Chocolate becomes a junk food.
- Chocolate creates obesity and diabetes.
- Causes acne, zits, blackheads (often a testosterone imbalance).
- Chocolate is addictive (people use it as a self-medicating food, like other sugar foods, salt foods, alcohol, etc.).
- Chocolate causes allergies – more likely the white sugars, nuts, milk – all con-

tained in store bought chocolates.

- Chocolate has no fiber – when processed it loses its fiber. We need both the soluble and the non-soluble fiber the seeds contain.
- Chocolate causes cavities. In actual fact, white sugar promotes acidity which increases bacteria that cause cavities. (For instance, sodas are a leading cause of cavities.)
- Chocolate causes migraines. It is actually the white sugar that does because it is toxic to the brain, not cacao.

Let's look at why a "food of the gods" healthy fruit became that bad.

As mentioned earlier, chocolate started out as just a seed or bean. The Aztecs and others began to add spices like chili peppers, vanilla, and various floral essences. The Spaniards added water. The English added the exotic raw sugars and then milk.

Subsequently, wax was introduced into the recipe, high fructose corn syrup, lecithin, vegetable oil, commercial shortening, etc.

Over time, chocolate recipes began to flourish and it did not take long before we had:

- A wide variety of chocolate-type candy bars.

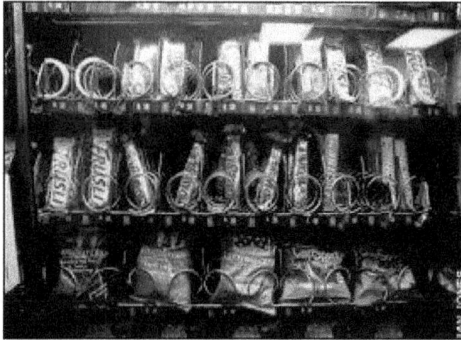

- Eventually we got more exotic brands like Lindt, Sprungli, Ghirardelli, Ferrero, Thornstons, Guylian, Godiva, Neuhaus, Richart, NOKA, Purdy's and more.

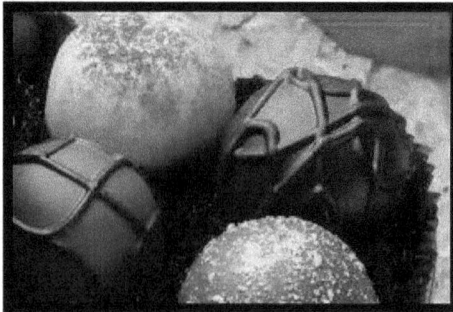

- We got dark, white, milk, caramel, pralines, truffles, fruit flavored, nut centered, soft centered, gel centered, soft chocolates, hard chocolates and more.
- We got the doughnuts – round, long, layered, with pieces, with toppings…

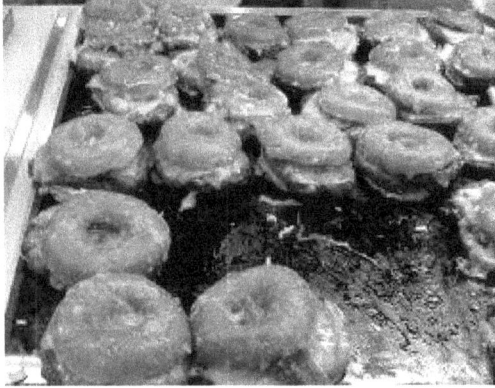

- Brownies, squares, cakes, pies, and my personal favorite, chocolate mousse!

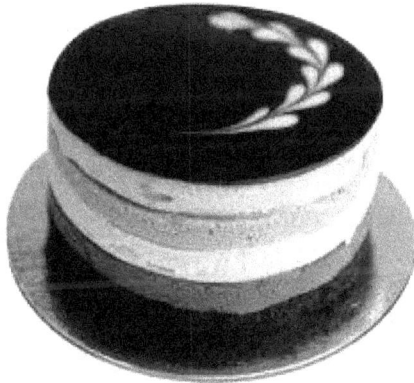

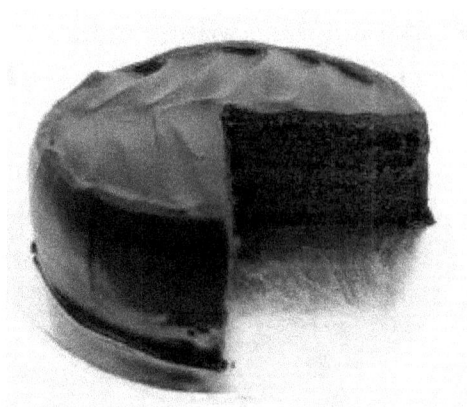

- Chocolate ice cream
- Various hot chocolate drinks

With all these variations of the chocolate seed, it is understandable that in 2008-2009 the world produced 3,515,000 tonnes of cocoa. This is equivalent to the weight of a line of double-decker buses stretching more than three times the length of Britain. Yes, we eat that much chocolate!

See:
http://www.kew.org/plants-fungi/Theobroma-cacao.htm

Chocolate became a comfort food, a treat/reward food and an indulgent food. So the problem evolved, that the more varied it became, the more processed it became, the more of a detriment it became. We created a monster out of a "food from the gods".

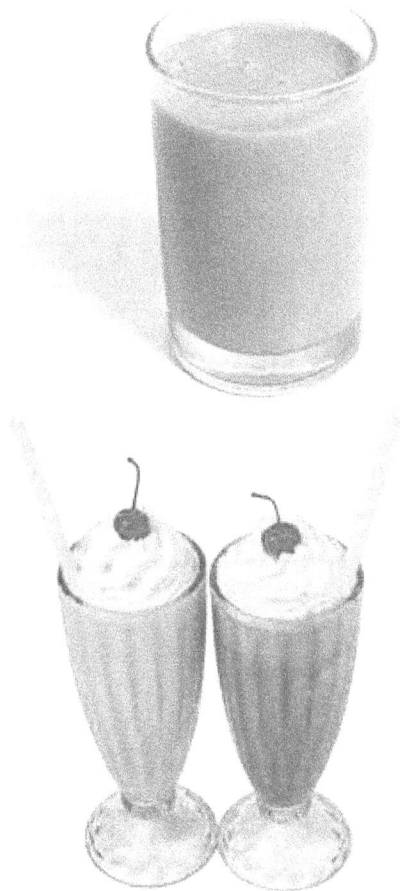

This new food monster was not only pasteurized (losing all of its nutrients) but, as noted, full of wax, high processed fructose corn syrup, stabilizers, preservatives, and a wide variety of additional artificial flavorings and other toxic chemicals.

This awesome food of the gods has become a contributor to:
- Obesity
- diabetes
- arteriosclerosis
- hypertension
- compromised gut
- compromised liver
- cavities
- headaches
- allergies

Oh, the poor chocolate gods! What they must be thinking...

It all goes to prove the point that the more man gets involved, the more toxic the food becomes.

But, there is good news. Let's keep reading.

SIX

What Nutrients in Chocolate make it Good for you?

The cacao fruit is the most pharmacologically complex, nutrient dense food source in the Amazon jungle. According to a variety of sources, it contains over 1200 individual chemical constituents comprising over 380 nutrients that our bodies require. All of that, is in chocolate.

In the last decade, these seeds have gone through extensive research and we are constantly finding out great, new, exciting information.

Because of all the research now being focused on foods (rather than artificial, synthetic, toxic pharmaceuticals), and because of all the different ailments that foods are shown to have an effect on chocolate is now coming to the center stage of a wide variety of institutions, associations and journals, such as:

Scientific Journals
- Journal of Nutrition
- Journal of American Medical Association
- International Journal of Obesity
- British Journal of Medicine
- Journal of the American College of Cardiology
- American Journal of Clinical Nutrition

Universities/Research Institutions
- Yale University
- Oxford University
- Harvard University
- University of Vienna
- Georgetown University
- University of Barcelona
- http://www.virginiaearl.myxocai.com/science-of-chocolate

(Note: Already this list is outdated because it is continually expanding.)

Here are a few examples of published articles:

- Journal of the American College of Cardiology, "Sustained Benefits in Vascular Function Through Flavanol-Containing Cocoa in Medicated Diabetic Patients".

• The American Journal of Clinical Nutrition, "Short-term administration of dark chocolate is followed by a significant increase in insulin sensitivity and a decrease in blood pressure in healthy persons".

• The Journal of Nutrition, "Blood Pressure is Reduced and Insulin Sensitivity Increased in Glucose-Intolerant, Hypertensive Subjects after 15 Days of consuming High-Polyphenol Dark Chocolate".

• Daily News Central, "Dark Chocolate Helps Counter Heart Damage from Smoking. Got Chocolate? Study Shows Its Heart-Healthy Chocolate Ingredient May Stop Cancer Cell Division".

• Medscape from WebMD, "Dark Chocolate May Improve Insulin Sensitivity/Resistance and Blood Pressure". UCDavis (University of California) "Heart-Healthy

Compound in Chocolate Identified".

- http://healthbychocolate.weebly.com/xocai-health.html

- Journal of Cerebral Blood Flow and Metabolism. "Researchers say they have identified the molecular mechanism by which a compound in cocoa can guard against the damage of a stroke".

- University of Califorina: UCDavis, "Heart Healthy Compound in Chocolate Identified".

- http://www.thefivereasons.com/Chocolate_and_Science.html

And the articles span a wide collection of topics. Here are a few of the arenas that scientists have researched with chocolate:

- Antioxidant properties (more than 250 studies)
- Cardiovascular health (more than 200)
- Diabetes (appx. 30 studies)

- Brain health (more than 60 studies)
- Mood (more than a dozen studies)
- Cell protective properties (more than 70 studies)
- Inflammation (appx. 40)
- Obesity (appx 25)
- Skin health (more than 30)

See:
http://www.virginiaearl.myxocai.com/science-of-chocolate

Again, these numbers are already outdated as there is an ever expanding list as the research continues.

Let's briefly look at a few of the nutrients in real chocolate to get an appreciation of why it is so good for you. This book will only review a few of the 380+ nutrients found in real chocolate.

MINERALS

Magnesium – an alkaline earth metal required for over 300 enzymes processes in every cell of your body:

- to make fuel - ATP;
- to make DNA and RNA; promotes muscle relaxation
- important to illnesses such as asthma, diabetes and osteoporosis because it facilitates calcium absorption

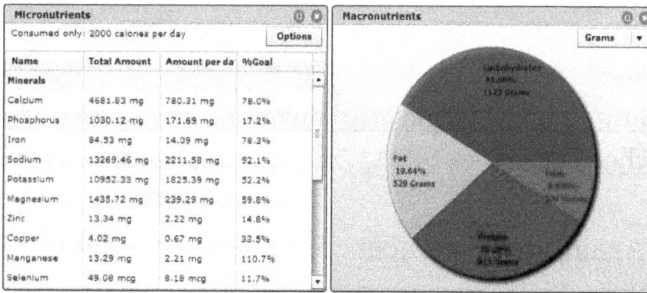

Name	Total Amount	Amount per da	%Goal
Minerals			
Calcium	4681.63 mg	780.31 mg	78.0%
Phosphorus	1030.12 mg	171.69 mg	17.2%
Iron	84.53 mg	14.09 mg	78.2%
Sodium	13269.46 mg	2211.58 mg	92.1%
Potassium	10952.33 mg	1825.39 mg	52.2%
Magnesium	1435.72 mg	239.29 mg	59.8%
Zinc	13.34 mg	2.22 mg	14.8%
Copper	4.02 mg	0.67 mg	33.5%
Manganese	13.29 mg	2.21 mg	110.7%
Selenium	49.08 mcg	8.18 mcg	11.7%

Calcium:
- important mineral for bone, nail, and hair health;
- provides a signaling function in many cell processes;
- neurotransmitter release;
- muscle contraction;
- electrical stimulation of the heart

Copper:
- facilitates absorption of iron;
- involved in growth;
- important in anti-oxidants;

- super oxide dismutase,
- hydrogen peroxide, etc.

Manganese:
- an important cofactor in a broad
- spectrum of enzymes;
- super oxide dismutase;

Phosphorous:
- important in the production/ transportation of fuel in the body - ATP;
- DNA & RNA, cellular membranes (phospholipids);
- bone and teeth enamel

Zinc:
- a trace element found in over 100 enzymes;
- in side chains of several amino acids;
- plays a key role in semen, prostate;
- helps regulate apoptosis (cell death);
- modulates brain activity

VITAMINS

B1 (Thiamine):
- energy, ATP, glycogenesis;
- necessary for a healthy CNS & mucous membrane

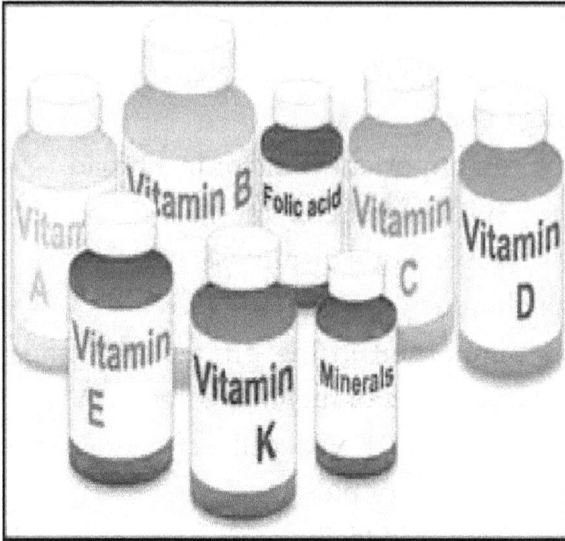

B2 (Riboflavine):

- energy, ATP, converts carbs into energy;
- metabolizes Vit A;
- synthesis of Vitamin B9;
- converts tryptophan to Vit B3;
- involved in glutathione redox

B3 (Niacin):

- energy, ATP,
- causes a decrease in free fatty acids -> VLDL cholesterol

B5 (Pantothenic acid):

- required to make CoA for Krebs Cycle/ATP;

- metabolize proteins, carbs and fats

B6 (Pyridoxine):

- amino acid metabolism;
- gluconeogenesis -> ATP
- sphingolipids: signalling in the brain and cell recognition

C:

- very high in Vitamin C; note: this is the entire Vitamin C and not just the anti-oxidant outer ring of ascorbic acid;
- co-factor for 8 enzyme processes to produce collagens (necessary for connective tissues: cartilage, tendon, ligaments, etc.)

K1:

- coagulation;
- treats warfarin toxicity

K2:

- bone formation : prevents liver/prostate cancer

SUGARS

Sugar, like fats, proteins and carbs, can be either good or bad. The body requires many sugars to make a wide variety of molecules. For instance, glycoproteins are sugar protein complexes that are involved in a wide variety of functions. Ribose is a particularly important sugar as it is the middle molecule in our fuel – ATP.

Coco sugar is good for diabetics: "A natural sweetener and functional food, coco sugar is a much welcome development for diabetics and hypoglycemics," said the Philippine Council for Agriculture, Forestry, and Natural Resources Research and Development (Pcarrd). Compared with refined cane sugar, coco sugar has a glycemic index (GI) at 35. ..much lower than the 54 GI, the level which nutritionists consider as safe for people who have to watch their glucose levels.

FIBER and FATS

Soluble fiber
  • slows blood glucose uptake in the liver (very good for diabetics)
Non soluble fiber
  • regulates colon function, transport;

(good for people who have challenges with bowel movements – either constipation or diarrhea)

Cocoa butter

- contains stearic acid – the most stable vegetable fats containing anti-oxidants that prevent rancidity
- Palmitic acid (regulates cholesterol)
- Oleic acid (prevents ALD, & reduces blood pressure),
- Linoleic acid

ANTI-OXIDANTS

- Polyphenols:
- Flavonoids (bioflavonoids) & Flavanols
- Anthocyanins & Catechins
- (procynides, proanthocyanins) (epicatechins)
  - Dr. Norman Hollenburg from Harvard Medical School believes that epicatechins are so important that they should be considered a vitamin

Cocoa 'Vitamin' Health Benefits Could Outshine Penicillin

ScienceDaily (Mar. 12, 2007) — The health benefits of epicatechin, a compound found in cocoa, are so striking that it may rival penicillin and anaesthesia in terms of importance to public health, reports Marina Murphy in Chemistry & Industry, the magazine of the SCI. Norman Hollenberg, professor of medicine at Harvard Medical School, told C&I that epicatechin is so important that it should be considered a vitamin.

The same Dr. Norman Hollenberg says "We all agree that penicillin and anaesthesia are enormously important. But epicatechins could potentially get rid of 4 of the 5 most common diseases in the western world, how important does that make epicatechin? I would say "very important" in diseases such as stroke, heart failure, cancer and Type 2 diabetes.

See:
http://chocolateandprosperity.net/latest_news

Real, cold-pressed chocolate, i.e., Xocai® chocolate, has 3-4 times the amount of epicatechins as acai berry, blueberry, and pomegranates and twenty times more anti-oxidants than green tea.

FLAVONOIDS

Another powerful group of polynutrients

- Alkalizes the body
- Anti-cancer
- Anti-bacterial
- Anti-inflammatory
- Anti-oxidant
- Anti-viral
- Act like hormones without damaging side effects
- Hypoglycemic
- Increases energy
- Lower risk of dementia
- Maintains mental function
- Prevents tooth decay
- Protect/repair the liver
- Reduces inflammation & chronic in-flammation
- Reduces oxidative stress
- Regulate platelets and coagulation
- Relieve allergy symptoms
- Slows aging

- Vaso-dilate /constrict blood arteries

THEOBROMINE

- Oil of Theobroma or Cacao Butter or Cocoa Butter; a yellowish white solid with the scent of Cacao
- excellent emollient properties (increase skin hydration) to soften and protect chapped hands and lips
- for inflammation of the liver or other organs
- mental stupor
- as a febrifuge (lowers fevers) especially in serious illnesses

See:
http://www.xocoatl.org/science.htm

PHARMACOLOGICALLY ACTIVE INGREDIENTS

See: http://www.xocoatl.org/science.htm

Below is a summary chart of an overview of nutritional values seen in a wide range of chocolates. The numbers are percentages of a given weight of chocolate.

Ingredient	Cocoa -low fat (European type)	Cocoa -high fat (Breakfast cocoa)	-Unsweetened chocolate	Bittersweet chocolate	Semisweet chocolate and baking chocolate
Fat	10-15%	20-25%	45-55%	33-45%	20-35%
Carbohydrates	45-60%	45-60%	30-35%	20-50%	50-70%
Sugars	0-2%	0-2%	0-2%	13-45%	45-65%
Dietary fibers	20-35%	30-35%	15-20%	5-8%	3-8%
Protein	17-22%	15-20%	10-15%	5-10%	3-8%
Calories per a oz	ca 60	ca 90	140-150	150-160	130-160
Calories per a 100 g	ca 200	ca 300	470-500	500-550	450-550

See: http://www.cacaoweb.net/nutrition.html

At this rate, one might want to replace their multi-vitamin/mineral tablets with chocolate.

SEVEN

So what is Chocolate good for?

So what is real Chocolate good for? We have already seen a wide selection of topics above but first, let's go over a few health issues and briefly explain each one. The following chapters will go into specific diseases and disorders in more detail.

We have to remember that commercial dark or bitter chocolate is not the same cold-pressed Xocai® chocolate.

Bitter or dark chocolate has been "dutch-pressed" to remove all the cocoa butter which is then sold at a high cost for white chocolate and other products. In the process, dutch-pressed chocolate has lost up to 80% of its rich anti-oxidants. This is particularly ironic considering that dark bitter chocolate is marketed on the basis of the anti-oxidants it supposedly provides.

Now, another ironic fact is that all chocolate is dark chocolate. Milk chocolate or light chocolate is only light because it has been pasteurized and had milk added to it. This may have been a good thing in the day when milk was raw and good for you. However, in today's world, milk has become just another processed product which, like other man-made products, is largely detrimental to your health.

Think back to the days, if you can, when you took milk from the cow to the fridge and it lasted 2 – 3 days. Now consider how long it has taken to get to the supermarket then off the shelf to you and how long it lasts in your fridge. Just like white bread that can last nearly forever, milk has nothing left in it to go bad, all so it has a long shelf life.

Xocai® chocolate has been independently laboratory tested to ensure that the patented process does in fact protect the nutrients. Xocai® Healthy Chocolate products are routinely tested and certified by Brunswick Laboratories and carry the Brunswick Labs Certified Seal.

Let's look at why real healthy chocolate, like Xocai® chocolate, is so good for you.

1) Great for Heart Health
- Lowers high blood pressure within 2-4 weeks
- Improves cardiovascular function
- Increases vaso-dilation
- Repairs inflamed arteries
- Reverses oxidized cholesterol
- Reduction of plaque

(See Chapter 8 for more information.)

2) Promotes weight loss (When eaten 30 min before a meal.)
- Fat cells release their toxins
- Regulates leptin and ghrelin
- Alters the DNA of fat cells into fatty acids for fuel

(See Chapter 9 for more information.)

3) Promotes sleep
- Enhances melatonin and dimethyltriptamine

4) Is very good for the gut

- Regulates acid production, i.e., acid reflux
- Full of polyphenol anti-oxidants that work with the immune system
- Subdues heart burn

(See Chapter 11 for more information.)

5) Safe for Type 2 diabetics
- Regulates blood glucose uptake
- Liver protection
- Pancreas protection

(See Chapter 10 for more information.)

6) Great for Depression
- Amino acids
- Neurotransmitters
- Anti-oxidants
- Natural anti-depressants
- Endorphins – feel good neurotransmitters
- Enhances cognitive function: memory, concentration, decision making, etc (University of Nottingham: increases blood flow to the brain)

7) Improves vision, skin, nails, dental health

(See Chapter 17 for more information.)

8) Histamine blocker
- reduces allergic reactions

(See Chapter 16 for more information.)

9) Coughing:
- A molecule called theobromine suppresses the vagus nerve (10th cranial nerve) which is responsible for coughing
- Professor Maria Belvisi reported "Not only did theobromine prove more effective than codeine, at the doses used it was found to have none of the side effects"

Real chocolate helps almost everything!

EIGHT

Chocolate and the Heart

Real chocolate is a food for the heart in more ways than one. We love the taste of chocolate and we love the benefits of chocolate. But do you know what chocolate does physiologically for the heart?

Because real chocolate provides a number of important benefits to the heart it has received the attention of the American Heart Association.

Just the anti-oxidant activity alone accomplishes the following:
- Reduces cardiac inflammation
- improves blood platelet function;
- decreases clotting;
- increases HDL, reduces LDL,
- increases prostacyclin (helps blood vessels to
- relax); effect stayed for 30 days

- reduces blood pressure
- reversed blood vessel damage
- lowers C-reactive protein levels (marker of cardiovascular disease risk)

(Archives of Internal Medicine (2007))

Harvard School of Public Health 140 studies: The principal fat in cocoa, stearic acid is metabolized differently than other fats and it should reduce cardiac conditions.

Journal of American College of Cardiology: 2008

In addition, the procyanidins do the following:

1. Procyanidins lower blood pressure by suppressing endothelin-1, a peptide that has an undesirable vasoconstriction effects. They also increase nitric oxide in the blood causing vasodilation and increased blood flow.

2. Procyanidins decrease platelet aggregation, thus preventing clot formation and blockage of arteries.

3. Procyanidins prevent oxidation of LDL-

cholesterol.

High blood cholesterol levels are a major risk factor for heart disease because LDL-cholesterol can accumulate in the artery wall where after oxidation it causes inflammation and the formation of plaque. When LDL-cholesterol is protected from oxidation it is less likely to cause atherosclerosis.

See: http://EzineArticles.com/4333961

Let's briefly review some of the studies:

1) Sustained Benefits in Vascular Function Through Flavanol-Containing Cocoa in Medicated Diabetic Patients

What this title is saying is that diabetic patients continue to experience heart benefits from the plant nutrients in chocolate for a prolonged period of time.

A Double-Masked, Randomized, Controlled Trial

Jan Balzer, MD[*], Tienush Rassaf, MD[*], Christian Heiss, MD[*], Petra Kleinbongard, PhD[*], Thomas Lauer, MD[*], Marc Merx, MD[*], Nicole Heussen, PhD[†], Heidrun B. Gross, PhD[‡], Carl L. Keen, PhD[‡], Hagen Schroeter, PhD[§] and Malte Kelm, MD[**] Department for Cardiolo-

gy, Pulmonology, and Vascular Medicine, University Hospital RWTH Aachen, Aachen, Germany

†*Department of Medical Statistics, University Hospital RWTH Aachen, Aachen, Germany*

‡*Department of Nutrition, University of California, Davis, California*

§*Mars Symbioscience, Rockville, Maryland.*

Goal: Does daily intake of the cocoa flavonoids improve heart function in medicated diabetic patients.

Conclusions: Diets rich in flavanols reverse vascular dysfunction in diabetes, highlighting therapeutic potentials in cardiovascular disease.

Translation: what this is saying is that diabetics can actually reverse dysfunction in the arteries and veins due to the particular type of flavonoid plant nutrients in chocolate.

http://content.onlinejacc.org/cgi/content/abstract/51/22/2141

2) Researchers Identify a Compound in Cocoa Responsible for Improving Blood Flow

Translation: People with hypertension have poor blood flow. A compound in chocolate resolves this issue.

Published today in the Proceedings of the National Academy of Sciences of the United States of America (PNAS)

Goal: Determine specific compounds present in cocoa and cardiovascular health

Conclusion: This new study identifies the flavanol, (-)epicatechin, as one of the bioactive nutrients in cocoa that can improve the ability of blood vessels to relax

Translation: The epicatechins in chocolate, which are powerful anti-oxidants, improve the arteries' ability to expand and contract, thus allowing for better blood flow and reducing hypertension.

3) Blood pressure is reduced and insulin sensitivity increased in glucose-intolerant, hypertensive subjects after 15 days of consuming high-polyphenol dark chocolate.

Translation: the plant nutrients in chocolate reduce hypertension and reverse diabetes.

Grassi D, Desideri G, Necozione S, Lippi C, Casale R, Properzi G, Blumberg JB, Ferri C.

Department of Internal Medicine and Public Health, University of L'Aquila, 67100 L'Aquila, Italy. davide.grassi@cc.univaq.it

Goals: Do cocoa flavanols increase nitric oxide bioavailability, protect vascular endothelium, and decrease cardiovascular disease (CVD) risk factors. (endothelial function, insulin sensitivity, beta-cell function, and blood pressure (BP) in hypertensive patients with impaired glucose tolerance (IGT))?

Conclusion: Flavanol-rich cocoa foods have a positive impact on CVD risk factors.

Translation: The type of flavonoids in chocolate increase the body's Nitric Oxide which improves the arteries capacity to expand and contract. Further, these flavonoids protect the membrane of the arteries and decrease risk of heart disease. Finally, these same flavonoids improve insulin sensitivity and impaired glucose intolerance in diabetics.

http://www.ncbi.nlm.nih.gov/pubmed/18716168?ordinalpos=1&itool=EntrezSystem2.PEntrez.Pubmed.Pubmed_ResultsPanel.Pubmed_DefaultReportPanel.Pubmed_RVDocSum

Arch Biochem Biophys. 2008 Aug 15;476(2):211-5. Epub 2008 Mar 6.

4) Do flavanols from cocoa lower vascular arginase activity in endothelial cells, i.e., lining of the arteries?

Translation: Cocoa lowers an enzyme (arginase) and raises a gas (nitric oxide) that improves the function of arteries.

Schnorr O, Brossette T, Momma TY, Kleinbongard P, Keen CL, Schroeter H, Sies H.

Institute for Biochemistry and Molecular Biology I, Building 22.03, Heinrich-Heine-University Duesseldorf, Universitaetsstrasse 1, D-40225 Duesseldorf, Germany. schnorr@uni-duesseldorf.de

Goal: Nitric Oxide (NO) is a key component in vasodilation – ability of the arteries to expand and contract. Increases in the enzyme: Argninase reduces levels of NO. Do cacao epicatechins help increase NO in double blind, cross over studies.

Conclusions: In both rats and humans, Flavonal rich Cacao drinks lowered arginase & increase NO.

Translation: Cocoa improves heart and blood function.

http://www.ncbi.nlm.nih.gov/pubmed/18348861?ordina lpos=5&itool=EntrezSystem2.PEntrez.Pubmed.Pubmed _ResultsPanel.Pubmed_DefaultReportPanel.Pubmed_R VDocSum

5) Heart-healthy Compound In Chocolate

Identified

ScienceDaily (Jan. 20, 2006) — "Although previous studies strongly indicated that some flavanol-rich foods, such as wine, tea and cocoa can offer cardiovascular health benefits, we have been able to demonstrate a direct relationship between the intake of certain flavanols present in cocoa, their absorption into the circulation and their effects on cardiovascular function in humans," said UC Davis biochemist Hagen Schroeter, who co-authored the paper along with cardiologist Christian Heiss of the Heinrich-Heine University.

Translation: Cocoa benefits cardiovascular functions.

http://chocolateandprosperity.net/latest_news

Harvard Health, February 2009, claimed that:

"Flavonoids are present in many healthful foods, like apples and cherries, but dark chocolate is the richest source. So it's no surprise that chocolate has attracted the interest of scientists from around the world, giving the research an international flavor. Most studies have concentrated on cardiovascular health; here are some representative findings:

Antioxidant activity. Among other beneficial actions, flavonoids protect LDL cholesterol from oxidation, which puts the "bad" into "bad cholesterol." Dark chocolate reduces LDL oxidation while actually increasing levels of HDL (good) cholesterol.

Endothelial function. The endothelium, the thin inner layer of arteries, is responsible for producing nitric oxide, a chemical that widens blood vessels and keeps their linings smooth. European studies have shown that dark chocolate improves endothelial function in healthy people. Further, that flavonoid-rich cocoa can reverse the endothelial dysfunction produced by smoking, and that dark chocolate may improve coronary artery function in heart transplant patients.

Blood pressure. Studies from Italy, Argentina, Germany, and the United States show that dark chocolate can lower blood pressure, though the effect is modest. The benefit wears off within a few days of stopping "treatment" with a daily "dose" of dark chocolate.

Blood clotting. Most heart attacks and many strokes are caused by blood clots that form in critical arteries. Researchers in Switzerland and the United States found that dark chocolate reduces platelet activation, a step in clot formation.

See:
http://www.health.harvard.edu/press_releases/The-health-benefits-of-that-heart-shaped-box-of-dark-chocolate

See:
http://journals.lww.com/cardiovascularpharm/Fulltext/2006/06001/The_Anti_inflammatory_Properties_of_Cocoa.10.aspx?WT.mc_id=HPxADx20100319xMP

It becomes easier and easier to see why real chocolate is so good for so many heart issues.

NINE

Chocolate and Weight Management

"No way!" you say? "Real chocolate eliminates weight?"

The answer is, yes, and it may amaze you. For example, chocolate has been shown to affect the following.

A) Gates or opens fat cells – to release toxins
B) Changes DNA so that lipids becomes a fatty acid – used for energy and eliminated
C) Balances the leptin and ghrelin hormones
D) Regulates genes involved in fat metabolism by restricting fat metabolism & storage;
E) Stimulates thermo genesis (fat burning)

Chocolate can also create obesity, diabetes, arteriosclerosis, headaches. You're probably thinking that this doesn't make sense.

Actually, it does make sense. Let's look at what

is going on here. When chocolate is pasteurized it loses all of its great nutrients, is combined with waxes and high fructose corn syrup, stabilizers, colorants, artificial and natural flavorings. (Note: All kinds of toxic chemicals can hide behind the label "natural flavorings".) By the time it has undergone all that processing, chocolate has become a source of toxins and is detrimental to the body.

But when chocolate is "clean" – processed at a very low heat – the protected nutrients have a wonderful impact on our general health and our weight management.

Here is why.

FATS

Water does not break down fat. Fat breaks down fat but it has to be good fats, like those found in foods like avocados, chocolate, olive oil and hemp seeds to work well.

If you remember in previous chapters we talked about the cocoa butter/liquor in chocolate. The types of fats in the cocoa butter are just the fats we need.

This is what WEBMD says about chocolate:
WebMD says chocolate is a Flat Belly Food

They're packed with monounsaturated fatty acids (also known as MUFAs, pronounced MOO-fahs). Those good-for-you fats protect you from chronic disease and, according to new research, can help you lose fat, specifically around your middle.

That's why they're at the heart of the Flat Belly Diet. There are five major categories of MUFAs: (1) oils, (2) nuts and seeds, (3) avocado, (4) olives, and (5) chocolate.

Now, what kind of fats do we have in cocoa butter?

1) Stearic acids
   • Correlated with lowered LDL cholesterol
2) Palmitic acids
   • Anti-oxidant
   • Helps prevent atherosclerosis
   • If combined with linoleic acid does not raise cholesterols

3) Capric acid (also in coconuts)
   - Medium chain fatty acid
   - Anti-microbial
   - Works against HIV, herpes simplex, chlamydia
4) Myristic acid (found in nutmeg)
   - Important to the phospholipids membrane around every cell
5) Arachidic acid
   - Important to the brain and eyes
6) Lauric acid (also in coconut oil)
   - medium chain fatty acid;
   - transforms into monolaurin – anti-microbial)
7) Oleic acid (also in olive oil)
   - Important to build brain cells
   - Important for the myelination of neurons
   - Reduces cholesterols
8) Linoleic acid
   - The foundation of the omega 6 fatty acids
   - Your brain needs both alpha linoleic and linoleic to make DHA and arachidic acid (AA).

See: http://www.healingdaily.com/detoxification-diet/coconut-oil.htm

See: http://www.fi.edu/learn/brain/fats.html

See: http://www.livestrong.com/article/521518-palmitic-acid-health-benefits/

Saturated fats	57-64%: **stearic acid** (24-37%), **capric acid** (0-10%), **myristic acid**, (0-4%), **arachidic acid** (1%), **lauric acid** (0-1%)
Unsaturated fats	36-43%
Monounsaturated fats	29-43%: (29-38% **oleic acid**, 35–41% **palmitoleic acid**),
Polyunsaturated fats	0-5% : (**linoleic acid**, 0–3%, 1-4%, **Linolenic acid** (0-1%)

Eating one serving of any of these foods at every meal will help reduce your accumulation of dangerous belly fat and control your calorie intake. You'll lose inches and pounds, too, especially around your waistline.

TOXINS

Our fat cells actually are very beneficial to us in that they help protect us from toxins in the body. Unfortunately, when the body has to compensate like this, there is always a reason for the compensation and there is always a cost involved.

The reason for the necessary compensation is that our liver is not functioning at full speed. Far to often, we are suffering from two problems in the liver:

1.) Non alcoholic fatty liver disease (NAFLD) – or some similar issue. The liver is the body's primary detoxifying organ and it is seriously overwhelmed with dealing with today's diets and lifestyles. The liver is responsible for over 500 functions that support every system, organ and process in the body.

2.) Deficient levels of glutathione. Considered to be the body's master anti-oxidant, glutathione is a million times more powerful than any of the dietary/supplement anti-oxidants. The highest concentration of it is in the liver.

So when one of the most important molecules

to the liver is deficient; the liver becomes ineffective; the toxins get released throughout the body and the fat cells struggle to help out by taking the toxins in.

We then start packing the weight on until we are not only way too heavy but now we are pre-diabetic. The domino effect continues as our health goes down the drain!

To the rescue comes real chocolate, not the pasteurized, waxy, high fructose corn syrup-laden "junk" chocolate candy that contributed to the problems in the first place but real, antioxidant rich, nutrient dense chocolate.

The real chocolate – unpasteurized, non-dutch-pressed, real chocolate does a number of things for us:

- It opens the fat cells to release the toxins
- It cleans up the toxins
- It turns the DNA of fat cells into fatty acids
- The body uses the fatty acids as fuel
- We get thinner – Yay!

HORMONES

All this is not all that real chocolate does for us. There are two extremely important food metabolizing hormones that, for most people, are out of balance. They are leptin and ghrelin. When these hormones are out of balance and we gain weight, the first thing that most people do is go on a reducing diet.

With most of the diets that people choose to try, leptin which stimulates satiation, and ghrelin which stimulates hunger, now become even more out of balance. When they are out of balance we gain weight, seemingly no matter what we do. Have you ever done well on a diet only to gain back more weight afterwards? That's probably the leptin and ghrelin imbalance at work in your system.

These hormones need to be in balance not only for food metabolism but for all the other functions in which they are involved.

For instance, ghrelin is involved in:
- Circulatory and nervous system
- Lipolysis regulation (breakdown of fats)
- Gastric motility (stool movement)

- Stimulates growth hormone in the anterior pituitary gland
- Plays a role in the hippocampus (short term to long term memory)
- Required for cognitive adaptation to changing environments
- Required for the process of learning
- Activates NO (nitric oxide) pathways in the endothelial layer of the arteries – thus reducing hypertension/high blood pressure.

Leptin is also involved in:
- Regulating energy intake/expenditure
- Like insulin, it is an adiposity sign
- Plays a part in the central nervous system
- In conjunction with amylin (another hormone, one that is released with insulin) – regulates fat specific weight loss
- Modulates T-cell activity in the immune system
- Modulates the immune response to atherosclerosis (thickening of blood vessel walls due to cholesterol and other types of plaque)

- Promotes angiogenesis (new blood vessels) by increasing vascular endothelial growth factor
- Regulates bone metabolism and therefore bone mass
- Down regulated by testosterone and increased by estrogen
- It used to be thought that only adipose tissue secreted leptin but it is now recognized that leptin is also secreted by ovaries, skeletal muscle, lower stomach, breasts, bone marrow, pituitary and liver.

Earlier we said that the benefits of real chocolate include the following:
- Opens the fat cells to release the toxins
- Cleans up the toxins
- Turns the DNA of fat cells into fatty acids
- The body uses the fatty acids as fuel
- We get thinner

Now we can also add:
- Regulates Leptin and Ghrelin

We know from before that real chocolate

- Alkalizes the body – helps weight loss
- Primary number one source of magnesium which is huge in weight loss
- Provides the anti-oxidants that help detox for weight loss
- Provides the fibers that help both the gut and the liver – which aids in weight loss.

So, now you know – real chocolate can really help you lose weight.

TEN

Chocolate and Diabetes

The belief over the last number of decades has been that chocolate contributes to the creation of diabetes. So, why are we now changing that construct and claiming that chocolate can eliminate diabetes? There are a number of reasons.

Diabetics are significantly low in anti-oxidants. Real chocolate is very high in the powerful anti-oxidants.

Diabetics have low levels of flavonoids to promote nitric oxide (an important gas that allows the arteries to expand). Real chocolate is very high in flavonoids.

Diabetics have low levels of anti-oxidants and in particular, the ones called epicatechins which not only mimic insulin but increase insulin receptor sensitivity. Real chocolate has high levels of these.

Diabetics have low levels of procyanidin, another powerful anti-oxidant, another huge source of anti-oxidants. Real chocolate has high levels.

Diabetics have low levels of fiber that regulate the uptake of sugars in the liver and prevent sugar spiking. Real chocolate has high levels of soluble fibers.

ANTI-OXIDANTS

It is well recognized today that diabetics are extremely deficient in anti-oxidants. Oxidation or free radical damage is more likely to occur when blood glucose/sugar levels are high. With this profile, damage occurs to the micro blood vessels. Other affects include neuropathy (pain in the nerves), edema (water in the tissues, like the ankles), nephropathy (kidney damage) and retinopathy (damage to the eyes).

It is also well recognized that natural, real chocolate has naturally high level of anti-oxidants. The challenge is that you have to eat the right kind of chocolate to get the benefit.

As explained earlier, typical dark/bitter chocolate that you buy off the shelf at the supermarket check-out lost most of its anti-oxidants when the cocoa butter was eliminated.

However, all of the Xocai® Healthy Chocolate products are routinely tested and certified by Brunswick Laboratories and carry the Brunswick Labs Certified Seal ensuring that you are eating chocolate rich in antioxidants and especially loaded with flavanols. The special patent protects all these natural anti-oxidants.

FLAVANOLS

Flavanols, plant compounds found in cocoa (as well as in tea, red wine, and certain fruits and vegetables), help blood vessels to function better and could help prevent cardiovascular disease. According to new research published in the June 2012 issue of the Journal of the American College of Cardiology (JACC). The full article can be found here:

http://www.naturalnews.com/023499.html

http://chocolateandprosperity.net/latest_news
David Grassi from the University of L'Aquila,

Italy claimed that "...flavanols may exert significant vascular protection because of their antioxidant properties and increased nitric oxide bioavailability...In turn, nitric oxide bioavailability deeply influences insulin-stimulated glucose uptake and vascular tone.

"These findings indicate that (real) dark chocolate may exert a protective action on the vascular endothelial also by improving insulin sensitivity."

http://inhumanexperiment.blogspot.ca/2011/01/dark-chocolate-reduces-blood-pressure.htmlndothelium

http://www.diabetesincontrol.com/index.php?option=com_content&view-article&id=2593

EPICATECHINS

In addition, to being a strong anti-oxidant, epicatechins mimic insulin action.

These flavonoids also increase the insulin release from the isolated Beta Langerhan cells in the pancreas.

See:
http://diabetes.diabetesjournals.org/content/33/3/291

In diabetic red blood cells, epicatechins cause an increase in acetylcholinesterase activity which is significantly low in diabetics. (Acetylcholine is a neurotransmitter that is released from one neuron and attaches to a receptor of another neuron. Epicatechins release the neurotransmitter from the second neuron and recycle it).

PROCYANIDIN

An interesting benefit of the cocoa procyanidin is again the prevention of spiking of blood sugars in the liver.

See:
http://www.sciencedirect.com/science/article/pii/S0899900707000147

Cocoa procyanidin improves glucose metabolism.

See:
http://www.ajcn.org/content/81/3/541.short

Cocoa procyanidin in diabetes prevents diabetes-induced cataract formation.

See:
http://ebm.rsmjournals.com/content/229/1/33.short

FIBERS

There are two types of fibers – soluble and non-soluble. Real chocolate contains both. The non-soluble fiber helps regulate the movement of stools. Too fast a movement (diarrhea) or too slow a movement (constipation) effects a large number of very important functions involving absorption and nutrient transformation that occurs in the intestines with the movement of the stools.

The soluble fiber, however, has a tremendous impact on the blood glucose uptake in the liver. In other words, it slows down the sugar impact on the liver thus preventing the spiking of the sugar in the liver that causes diabetes.

Very simply, for people with diabetes, indulging in cocoa could be a way to improve their health naturally – and deliciously.

It sure makes sense why real chocolate will benefit diabetics, doesn't it? And on top of that, as noted from the last chapter...it aids in weight loss.

How much better can it get?

ELEVEN

Chocolate and the Gut

How can chocolate possibly be good for the gut?

Once again, you have to determine the difference between good and bad chocolate. Regular chocolate candy is junk food and extremely harmful to the gut. Along with other junk foods like sodas, micro-waved food, processed foods, chips, cookies, etc., chocolate junk is full of sugars and various other toxins that do damage to the lining of the gut, to the necessary microbes in the gut and to the immune system in the gut.

Yeast infections and other gut disorders will crave the regular pasteurized sugar filled chocolates to maintain the acidic environment and provide the sugars that they require to thrive on.

However, good, real chocolate will benefit the healthy gut in a number of different ways. Let's find out how.

The gut, or gastro-intestinal tract, holds about 90% of the body's immune system. The flavanols found in real chocolate support this immune system, support the molecules in the immune system and provide the micro/macro-pre/pro-biotics to keep the system functioning.

In addition, the alkalizing minerals, vitamins, amino acids, and all of polyphenols found in real chocolate provide the required good healthy nutrients that create a domino effect through the gut to maintain great health.

Of particular interest are the micro/macro-, pre/pro-biotics in real chocolate. In fact, Xocai® chocolate has a product called XBiotic® which is loaded with these wonderful, necessary nutrients.

Dark chocolate reduces the urinary excretion of stress hormones (like cortisol and catecholamines) and partially normalized stress-related gut microbial activities.

See:
http://www.ncbi.nlm.nih.gov/pubmed/19810704
And:
http://pubs.acs.org/doi/abs/10.1021/pr900607v

Do you think that real chocolate might benefit your gut?

TWELVE

Chocolate and Bone Density

It appears that we have a serious misunderstanding of bone density and its connection to calcium, not to mention the role of real chocolate in bone health. Let's start by taking a look at the role of calcium in our bodies.

CALCIUM

Calcium is required for a number of different functions in the body. The parathyroid monitors our blood to determine whether we need more or less free-floating calcium. If we need more calcium then the parathyroid sends out a hormone to the bones to metabolize or "turn over" thus releasing more calcium.

If we have enough calcium then the parathyroid hormone is not sent out. The bones slow down their metabolism and life continues.

However, we have heard through the media over the past few decades that we are all deficient in calcium. There is some logic to this rational as we know that we consume a lot of calcium-leaching foods such as soy milk, tofu, coffee, soda, alcohol, white flour, processed meats, and bran. In addition, pasteurization destroys calcium in many foods. We then have to take calcium tablets to make up for this deficiency.

Do you see the problem that occurs with this kind of process? We have now introduced calcium into the blood thereby telling the parathyroid that we have plenty of calcium. The parathyroid stops telling the bones to metabolize. Now we are creating more of a problem than we started with.

In addition, several minerals are required for bone metabolism. Calcium throws the balance of potassium, manganese, silica, phosphorous, magnesium, boron, Vitamin K2, and more, out of whack.

If what we need is not more calcium then what do we need? The answer is strontium. Strontium draws in all the minerals, and in balance, so that the bones do the work they are meant to do.

Instead, we were taught to take calcium, throw the messaging system out in the parathyroid, throw the balance of minerals out in the bones and we end up with a huge problem.

Next, we end up in the MD's office. Your doctor recognizes that you are low in calcium and provides you with medications. What do these medications do? They create even more of a problem!

The osteoporosis medications block the clean-up cells in the bones. These clean up cells are called osteoclasts. The medications, in effect, paralyze the osteoclasts from functioning. So now, our bones are plugged with all the garbage they needed to get rid of. So yes, we have dense bones but they are dense with left over waste and garbage which does us no good at all.

Now, there is another side to this complex issue. The 25% of postmenopausal women with the highest bone mass are 2.5 – 4 times more likely to be diagnosed with breast cancer than those with the lowest bone mass.

Apparently, hormones which maintain bone mass inadvertently create a higher breast cancer risk. In addition, women who take estrogen/hormone replacement still experience bone changes and often suffer breakages.

Currently, there is controversy about the bone mass density index, the test and the interpretation of the results.

See:
http://www.drmcdougall.com/misc/2012nl/jan/fav5.htm

During menopause, bones slow down production of new cells and tend to ignore the presence of calcium. When the reproductive system moves past menopause, so does this "bone pause". The bones rebuild themselves, especially if the appropriate nutrients are available. Dr. Campbell, Professor of Nutritional Biochemistry at Cornell University, made the following claim: "The closer people get to a diet based on plant foods and leafy vegetables, the lower the rates of many diseases, including osteoporosis." Women who consume lots of calcium-rich plants and exercise moderately build strong flexible bones. Women who rely on hormones build bones that are massive, but rigid.

So now what do we do?

CHOCOLATE – to the rescue!

So how does real chocolate fit into this equation? Well let's see.

First of all, junk food chocolate will continue to exacerbate the problem, whatever it is. The sugars cause an acidic environment and increase free radicals. Bone cannot metabolize in an acidic environment and the free radicals cause a lot of damage.

Real chocolate, however, has a huge benefit to bone metabolism.

1) Flavonoids:

a. reduce oxidative stress
b. reduce inflammation and chronic inflammation
2) Alkaloids: theobromine, phenthylamine
3) Alkalizing minerals: Magnesium
    a. about 50% of magnesium is stored in our bones
    b. magnesium helps regulate blood sugar levels
    c. promotes healthy blood pressure
    d. supports energy metabolism
    e. supports protein synthesis
    f. all of which is very helpful in bone metabolism
4) Minerals: Calcium, iron
5) Sugar: Real chocolate doesn't have high-fructose corn syrup or other toxic sugars
6) Oxalic acid: Some people will argue that real chocolate is actually detrimental because of the oxalic acid but the levels are such that it has negligible effect on calcium metabolism

PREVENTION OF OSTEOPOROSIS

Osteoporosis is diagnosed when bone mineral

density declines. This decline increases the risk for fractures. Women who consume greater amounts of antioxidants, for instance, like those found in dark, real chocolate, have higher bone mineral density levels than those who consume lower levels. This makes dark, real chocolate a great addition to the diet in anyone with low bone density or susceptibility to fracture.

See:

http://www.menopause-metamorphosis.com/An_Excerpt-103-better_bones.htm

Do you think your bones might benefit from you eating real chocolate?

THIRTEEN

Chocolate and Cancer

Even when I was a child, cancer had a bad reputation. It was whispered in company like a four letter word. It was scary and put everyone into a panic.

By the time I was twenty years old, I had witnessed the slow agonizing death of several people diagnosed with cancer. It was always a sad and difficult experience for everyone involved.

Then I was diagnosed with ovarian cancer myself. On a Friday afternoon, a tiny, Asian female oncologist hustled into the "patient room" where I waited. I was wearing one of those little white covers everyone had to wear back then. She simply told me that the big blotch that I had asked about on the ultrasound was in fact cancer and had to be removed immediately. I was told to make arrangements for surgery at the front desk and she would see me Monday morning! And she was gone. I stood there in shock and amazement, too stunned even to get dressed. I am not sure how long it took me to get changed and leave but eventually I found my way to the parking lot – apparently still in a daze as my husband was honking the car horn and waving at me to find where he'd parked.

He took one look at me. "What happened?" he said. "It looks like you have seen a ghost." I told him what the doctor had said to me. Shocked, we both sat there and stared out the front car window.

Eventually, I suggested that he take me to see my mother. If nothing else, it gave him something to do.

My mother was a librarian at the time and when I walked into her office, she said, "What happened? It looks like you have seen a ghost." Hadn't I just heard that? I must look pretty bad, I thought. I told her what the physician had said. "Do you want it?" she asked me.

What the heck kind of question was that? Of course I didn't want it. Was she crazy?

She repeated her question. "Do you want it?" Frustrated, I answered, "Well, of course, I don't!"

"Well then, get rid of it." It sounded to me like she thought I was some kind of idiot. If you don't want, get rid of it. What was so hard with that?

I thought she meant go home and get your body to get rid of it. What she really meant was to have the surgery and get rid of it.

I went home and phoned my osteopath-naturopath who had come out of retirement for the third time. He was in his eighties. He asked me a number of questions that I had no idea how to answer and then simply said, "Well, let's go on a betalaine diet."

He explained what I needed to do. My husband was wonderfully cooperative and went on it with me. And voila, in three and half weeks when I succumbed to the family pressure and went back in for another laparoscopy, there was no cancer!

I had lost the fear and dread of cancer. Since then I have worked with many people who have been diagnosed with cancer. I have learned what protocols work with which cancers.

There are so many treatments around the world with a huge number of scientific studies behind them. Unfortunately, here in North America we are not given the chance to work with these treatments.

Pharmaceutical companies control the oncologists – not only with what they learn but with what their options are. People often choose not to do their own research, often because their fear simply paralyzes them and/or they don't know where to look. They end up becoming victims of the system.

Now, you ask, what does that have to do with chocolate? How does chocolate play into this subject?

Let's look at some of the nutrients in real chocolate and find out how these nutrients interact with cancer cells.

In summary, real chocolate polyphenols do the following:

1) Turn on cell death in cancer cells (apoptosis)
2) Alter the cell membrane to let in oxygen rather than sugar (potentiation)
3) This creates an alkaline environment in the cell rather than acidic
4) Starve the cancer cells by blocking the development of new blood vessels (angiogenesis) and the nutrients they bring into the cells.

More specifically, we can look at the ingredients in real chocolate and understand what each group does:

Epicatechins :

- a form of catechin
- a natural powerful phenol antioxidant
- catechin interacts with a variety of human genes, for instance, CASP3 which turns on apoptosis (apoptosis means automatic preprogrammed cell death – this is turned off in cancer cells)

Procyanidins:
A type of condensed tannin in the polyphenol/ flavonoid category
- a natural anti-oxidant
- highly bioavailable
- low toxicity
- induce apoptosis (preprogrammed cell death)
- reduce androgen-dependent tumor growth
- plays a part in estrogen driven cancers
- reduce risk of cancer such as:
- cutaneous carcinoma,
- oral carcinoma
- breast carcinoma
- bronchogenic carcinoma
- liver carcinoma
- prostate carcinoma

- pancreatic carcinoma
- gastric carcinoma

See:
http://ezinearticles.com/?Wine-and-Health-Research---The-Power-of-Procyanidins---The-Real-French-Paradox&id=4333961

See: ttp://EzineArticles.com/4333961

- influences platelet function
- also works as anti-depressants and has MAOIs (Monoamine oxidase inhibitors) properties
- genes that promote cellular division
- that promote angiogenesis

See:
http://www.cancerletters.info/article/S0304-3835(01)00731-5/abstract

Anthocyanins:
- accelerate apoptosis – cell death
- prevent development of new arteries to absorb nutrients (angiogenesis)
- minimize DNA damage – new cells are not cancerous

Proanthocyandins:

- inhibits cancer growth by increasing different enzymatic processes
- allowing more oxygen into the cancer cells and increasing the alkalinity
- (Molecular Cancer Therapeutics : 2005)
- Georgetown University; Weill Cornell Medical College; Strang Cancer Prevention Center; Brigham & Women's Hospital; Journal of the American College of Cardiology 2008)

See: http://ezinearticles.com/?Wine-and-Health-Research---The-Power-of-Procyanidins---The-Real-French-Paradox&id=4333961

See: http://phys.org/news185087626.html

See: http://www.dailymail.co.uk/health/article-2091627/Eating-chocolate-stave-bowel-cancer-say-scientists.html
See: http://cancerbattlefield.com/functional-food/chocolate-your-life/

I would not suggest that you only use chocolate to get rid of cancer cells but you certainly can understand why I suggest people make it a part of their protocol. For one thing, it is a lot more fun to take than pills, tinctures, chemotherapy and radiation.

FOURTEEN

Chocolate and Depression

Depression is a complex process. Most researchers have long recognized that low serotonin levels play a very small part in depression. Yet anti-depressants are designed on the hypothesis that low serotonin causes depression.

More recently, pharmaceutical companies have also included synthetic artificial chemicals that alter levels of norepinephrine and dopamine. Why? Because the research shows the anti-depressants that regulate serotonin work for less than 40% of the population, less than 60% of the time. This works out to less than 24% of the time. To put that in perspective, the placebo effect is usually between 35-38%!

I worked as a psychologist for the past 20+ years and found that a lot of people did not have psychological issues yet suffered depression. This did not make sense according to all the theories I had been taught.

Since I have never stopped studying, I started to collect a lot of different ideas about how and why depression can evolve. Eventually, I got the opportunity to attend a Naturopathic School and started to study all the different physiological components that caused depression.

Here is a short list of physiological issues that can cause depression:
1) Compromised liver (huge numbers of patients have a compromised liver by the time they are 30)
2) Hypothyroid (a misunderstood concept)
3) Adrenal fatigue (most women today have adrenal fatigue)
4) Leaky gut syndrome
5) Fatty acid deficiency
6) Vitamin Bs deficiency
7) Glutathione deficiency
8) Anti-oxidant deficiency
9) Oxidative stress and inflammation:

a. Gut
b. Liver
c. Brain

How does real chocolate fit into all of this? Well, let me count the ways.

1) Real chocolate has the necessary fatty acids:
   a. for the brain
   b. for inflammation.
2) Real chocolate has B vitamins.
3) Real chocolate supports glutathione.
4) Real chocolate has a load of anti-oxidants.
5) Real chocolate provides the amino acids for neurotransmitter production, for instance, taurine, tryptophan.
6) Real chocolate has endorphins.
7) Real chocolate has anadamide – the "blissful" neurotransmitter.
8) Real chocolate actually has dopamine, a neurotransmitter, in it.
9) Real chocolate has natural anti-depressants called MAOIs (as an artifical synthetic drug, these are dan-

gerous but as a natural component of a healthy food they are great).

10) Real chocolate contains arginine – natural sexual stimulant.

11) Real chocolate has theobromine, a caffeine like molecule that stimulates CNS (cousin to caffeine – w/o the same side effects).

12) When real chocolate is consumed, it triggers the production of endorphins in the body which create a feeling of happiness.

13) Real chocolate contains phenylethylamine (PEA) love chemical which increases endorphins.

Many people eat when they are depressed. When this group of depressed patients was studied, the comfort foods they tended to eat contained the amino acids to make the neurotransmitters. That means that eating real chocolate when you are depressed makes sense.

If you are depressed, real chocolate might be a good thing to add to your diet. Just remember, junk chocolate will create more of a problem. You have to get the good stuff.

See:
http://www.chocolate-for-health.com /Depression.html

See:
http://www.webmd.com/balance/stress-management/news/20091113/dark-chocolate-takes-bite-out-of-stress

See:
http://www.everydayhealth.com/depression-pictures/8-foods-that-fight-depression.aspx#/slide-8

FIFTEEN

Chocolate and Inflammatory Diseases

Inflammatory diseases are not fun. They are painful.

Most people think of arthritis when they think of inflammatory disease but in today's world a large percentage of disease, disorder and dysfunction is related to free radicals becoming oxidative stress which in turn creates inflammation.

Flavonoid compounds in real chocolate exert strong anti-inflammatory effects by inhibiting the same enzyme that is the target of over-the-counter drugs such as ibuprofen and naproxen but without the negative toxicity that comes from taking artificial, synthetic drugs.

Before we go further, let me tell you another story. I used to suffer from osteo- and rheumatoid arthritis and fibromyalgia. At the time, I owned and operated several multi-million dollar businesses which may have contributed to my problems. I was in a lot of pain.

At one point, I was taking 3 to 4 Tylenol 3 with Codeine tablets, three or four times per day just to keep going. When I finally decided that I had had enough I started to do my own research. Although it took me a couple of years, I entirely eliminated all the pain and inflammation. Since then I have worked with numerous people who would rather eliminate their arthritis rather than simply manage it.

I wish I had known about real chocolate when I was suffering. As has been mentioned several times in this book, real chocolate is full of anti-oxidants, anti-inflammatories and all kinds of other nutrients that help with inflammatory conditions. Let's take a look at a few of them.

A subgroup of Polyphenols is called flavonoids. One of the most potent groups of these flavonoids are called epicatechins. Real chocolate is loaded with nutrients. Epicatechins are anti-oxidants. (They restore the free radicals and make them function in a healthy way.)

Real chocolate is also full of Omega 3 fatty acids which are well known anti-inflammatories.

Real chocolate is full of alkalizing minerals which aid in eliminating inflammation and oxidative stress.

Can you see why you might want to add real chocolate to your management or elimination of arthritis strategy?

References:
American Journal of Clinical Nutrition 2005:
- epicatechins and other flavanols inhibit leukotrienes – inflammatory mechanisms;
- flavanols inhibit COX-2, inflammatory cytokines and interleukin – 1beta

See:
http://www.drweil.com/drw/u/ART02012/anti-inflammatory-diet

See:
http://www.chronic-inflammation.com/natural-anti-inflammatory.html

See:

http://www.naturalremediesforbetterhealth.com/darkchocolate.html

See:

http://onlinelibrary.wiley.com/doi/10.1002/mnfr.200700435/abstract

See:

http://journals.lww.com/cardiovascularpharm/Fulltext/2006/06001/The_Anti_inflammatory_Properties_of_Cocoa.10.aspx?WT.mc_id=HPxADx20100319xMP

SIXTEEN

Chocolate and Autoimmune Diseases

There are a number of autoimmune disease that share similar deficiencies. Lupus, colitis, arthritis, eczema, chronic fatigue syndrome and so on, actually share common nutrient deficiencies.

Let's look at what they have in common and then why real chocolate might be part of the solution.

Common deficiencies shared by autoimmune diseases are:
- Theobrominine
- Tyramine
- Tryptophan
- Endorphins
- Anandamide
- Anti-oxidants

Interestingly enough, these substances are all

contained in real chocolate.

What do these nutrients do? Well, very simply, they address:

- inflammation
- pain
- Energy levels
- anxiety

Let's look at these in more detail.

Theobromine, aka xantheose

- A bitter alkaloid
- Highest amount found in Theobroma cacao
- Same family as caffeine, lesser effect on the central nervous system
- Vasodilator (promotes arteries to expand)
- Diuretic (increases urine production)
- Heart stimulant

Tyramine

- Derived from the amino acid tyrosine
- Acts as a catecholamine (dopamine, norepinephrine, epinephrine)

- Blood pressure regulation – vasocon-strictor

Tryptophan
- An essential amino acid
- Used in structural or enzyme proteins
- Required for neurotransmitters seroto-nin, melatonin, niacin,
- A metabolite is 5HTP which metabolizes into serotonin in the liver
- Degrades in auto-immune diseases

Endorphins
- Opioid peptides that function as neuro-transmitters
- Released during exercise, pain, con-sumption of spicy food, love, orgasm
- Triggered by acupuncture, floating

Anandamide
- A neurotransmitter related to bliss, de-light
- Converts to arachidonic acid (cycle): important to the cell's phosphilipid membrane
- regulate inflammation
- vaso-dilation of arteries

- regulation of platelets
- regulate calcium movement
- control hormone regulation
- control cell growth
- required for kidney function
- and much, much more
- abundant in the brain, muscles, and liver
- Involved in cellular signaling (communication)

Anti-oxidants
- Nutrients that are able to stabilize free radicals
- that cause so much damage to the body
- Abundant in real chocolate

You can imagine if all of these functions are distorted, reduced, or compromised that autoimmune diseases are a definite risk.

Yet, all of these nutrients are found in real chocolate.

References:
http://www.ncbi.nlm.nih.gov/pubmed/17611712

See:
http://onlinelibrary.wiley.com/doi/10.1002/mnfr.
200700435/abstract

See: http://www.superfood-
guru.com/autoimmunediseases.html

See:
http://en.wikipedia.org/wiki/Prostacyclin#Functi
on

See:
http://www.sciencedirect.com/science/article/pii
/S088915911100047X
www.plosone.org/.../info:doi%2F10.1371%2Fjourn
al.pone.0008688

See:
http://www.bellaonline.com/articles/art20258.as
p

SEVENTEEN

Chocolate and your Skin

You can understand how the seed of a fruit can have a complex array of nutrients that can impact a large number of issues in the body.

But the skin?

Journal of Nutrition (May, 2006) claimed that researchers found that certain components in cocoa may actually help improve the appearance of women's skin by increasing hydration, decreasing skin roughness and scaling and helping to support the skin's defense against UV damage.

The German scientists attributed the observed benefits to cocoa flavanols - a group of compounds that can be particularly rich in cocoa and that have been previously reported to improve blood flow and vessel function.

See:
http://chocolateandprosperity.net/latest_news

Apparently, the flavonoids which are also anti-oxidants leave the skin feeling smoother and moister. Further, they found that those who drank the cocoa showed less inflammation and/or redness in response to exposure to UV light. Most flavonoids absorb UV light.

See:
http://www.sciencenews.org/view/generic/id/7437/title/Food_for_Thought_Chocolate_as_Sunscreen

Real chocolate has been shown to make the skin:
- 16% denser
- 11% thicker
- 13% moister
- 30% less rough
- 42% less scaly

Nutrition has a tremendous impact on the skin and flavonoids are skin protectors. Vitamin A, Vitamin C, beta-carotene (and other carote-noids) and Vitamin E have all been shown to prevent sun damage and improve skin texture.

See:
http://www.bastyrcenter.org/content/view/1135

In addition, German researchers have also found that these same flavonoids can fight skin cancer.

See:
http://www.scribd.com/doc/80513372/Recent-Dark-Chocolate-Research-Studies-Show-That-%E2%80%9CCocoa-Solids-and-Flavonoids%E2%80%9D-Can-Fight-Off-the-Devastating-Effects-of-Skin-Cancer-%E2%80%93-Review-Xocai%E2%80%99s-H

All these nutrients are found in real chocolate.

EIGHTEEN

Chocolate and Alzheimer's

Numerous issues have been correlated with Alzheimer's disease. Once again, the process by which free radicals become oxidative stress, which in turn cause inflammation, has been associated with Alzheimer's disease.

Anti-oxidants

The brain uses 20% of the body's oxygen and therefore is at high risk for reactive oxygen species or free radicals. Consequently, the brain requires more anti-oxidants than most other parts of the body. The liver is probably the only organ that supersedes the brain.

Oxidative stress induced by reactive oxygen species (free radicals) has been strongly associated with the development of neurodegenerative disorders, including Alzheimer's disease.

We have already acknowledged that real chocolate leads all other foods in its anti-oxidant content. Thus, with regard to this issue alone, real chocolate is enormously beneficial to the brain and Alzheimer's.

In particular, the cocoa procyanidin fraction (CPF) and procyanidin B2 (epicatechin-(4_-8)-epicatechin) – all major polyphenol in cocoa – protect the brain, the neurons and the neuronal cells.

See:
http://pubs.acs.org/doi/abs/10.1021/jf0735073

See:
http://jn.nutrition.org/content/139/1/120.short

Fatty Acids

The brain is made up of almost 70% fatty acids. Fats make up about 70% of the insulation required on neurons. Oleic acid, found in real chocolate, makes up the majority of the myelination/insulation on the neurons.

Other fats in the brain include DHA and AA.

Crucial to the development of the brain and the eyes during fetal development, it continues to be important to the brain throughout our lives.

In addition, we require EFAs (essential fatty acids) like ALA (Alpha-linoleic acid) and LA (Linoleic acid).

See:
http://www.fi.edu/learn/brain/fats.html#fatsbuild

The fatty acids in real chocolate include:
- Stearic acids
- Palmitic acids
- Capric acid
- Myristic acid
- Arachidic acid
- Lauric acid
- Oleic acid
- Linoleic aicd

Do you think real chocolate might provide some nutrients for the brain, and in particular, for Alzheimer's sufferers?

Choline is also important to the brain. It is the basis for various nutrients involved in memory and brain function.

- Acetylcholine – neurotransmitter
- SAMe – fights depression
- Phosphotydalcholine – membrane sheath
- Sphingomyelin – membrane sheath

Although the body can make small amounts of choline, the majority of choline needs to be absorbed through food.

Real chocolate contains over 115mg of choline per
100 grams/3o mg/2 tablespoons of Real chocolate.

See: http://www.livestrong.com/article/84483-foods-rich-choline/
See http://www.diet.com/g/choline

Theobromine

The theobromine that we have already said is part of the real chocolate profile not only lowers blood pressure but inhibits beta-secretase.

Beta secretase is an enzyme that produces "beta amyloid" in the brain plaques typical of Alzheimer's disease.

What this means is that real chocolate protects the brain from Alzeheimer's.

See:
http://junebergalzheimers.com/index.php?option=com_content&view=article&id=183&Itemid=311

Do you want to protect your brain with real chocolate? Who wouldn't?

Appendix

It is difficult to keep up with all the exciting news and all of the peer-reviewed medical studies showing how high-flavanol cocoa could help your health.

Recently Xocai® was awarded with the United States government's acknowledgement of being the "Healthy Chocolate".

All of the Xocai® Healthy Chocolate products are routinely tested and certified by Brunswick Laboratories and carry the Brunswick Labs Certified Seal ensuring that you are eating chocolate rich in antioxidants and especially loaded with flavanols.

See:
http://chocolateandprosperity.net/latest_news

References:

- http://archive.fieldmuseum.org/chocolate/history.htm
- http://archive.fieldmuseum.org/chocolate/history_european9.htm l
- http://archive.fieldmuseum.org/chocolate/history_intro.html
- http://www.athenapub.com/chocolat.htm
- http://www.cacaoweb.net/cocoa-chocolate.html
- http://www.mythinglinks.org/ip~cacao.ht ml
- http://www.nhm.ac.uk/research-uration/research/projects/sloane-herbarium/hanssloane.htm
- http://www.livestrong.com/article/521518 -palmitic-acid-health-benefits/#ixzz1s9kbuZRk
- http://www.xocoatl.org/science.htm
- http://www.livestrong.com/article/459242 -cocoa-insulin-resistance/#ixzz1sB18gzpi

- "Dictionary of Nutraceuticals and Functional Foods"; N.A.M. Eskin; 2006
- "Journal of Medicinal Food": "Monoacylglycerol (MAG)-oleic Acid has Stronger Antioxidant, Anti-atherosclerotic, and Protein

Glycation Inhibitory Activities Than MAG-palmitic Acid"; K.H. Cho et al.; February 2010

- "Asian Pacific Journal of Clinical Nutrition": Cholesterolaemic Effect of Palmitic Acid in Relation to Other Dietary Fatty Acids"; M.A. French et al.; November 2002

- "American Journal of Clinical Nutrition"; Short-term Administration of Dark Chocolate Is Followed by a Significant Increase in Insulin Sensitivity and a Decrease in Blood Pressure in Healthy Persons; Davide Grassi, et al.; March 2005

- "Hunger hormone tied to learning". http://www.the-scientist.com/news/display/23132/. Retrieved 2007-06-01. at The Scientist

- Howard AD, Feighner SD, Cully DF, Arena JP, Liberator PA, Rosenblum CI, Hamelin M, et al. (1996). "A receptor in pituitary and hypothalamus that functions in growth hormone release". Science 273 (5277): 974-7

www.ingramcontent.com/pod-product-compliance
Lightning Source LLC
Chambersburg PA
CBHW070757290326
41931CB00011BA/2055